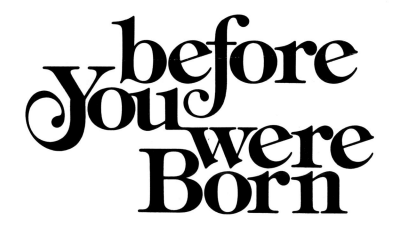

ISBN: 0-87973-353-5 (Hardbound Edition)
ISBN: 0-87973-343-8 (Paperbound Edition)

Library of Congress Catalog Card Number: 79-91741

Published, printed, and bound
in the United States of America

before you were Born

BY JOAN LOWERY NIXON

ILLUSTRATED BY JAMES McILRATH

Our Sunday Visitor, Inc.
Huntington, Indiana 46750

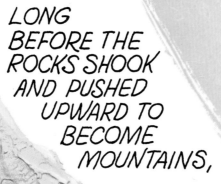

LONG BEFORE THE ROCKS SHOOK AND PUSHED UPWARD TO BECOME MOUNTAINS,

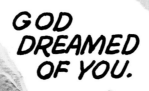

GOD DREAMED OF YOU.

AND BEFORE
THE SUN
WHIRLED HOT
INTO THE
DESERTS, AND
THE WIND
RUSHED COOL
INTO THE
VALLEYS,

**GOD
LOVED
YOU.**

EVEN BEFORE
THE EARTH
WAS CREATED,
GOD WANTED YOU
TO BE BORN.

**HE DREAMED OF YOU.
HE LOVED YOU. HE WANTED YOU.**

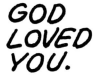

WHEN YOUR LIFE BEGAN YOU WERE SO SMALL NO ONE KNEW YOU WERE THERE.
EXCEPT GOD.
FAR AWAY, THE TINIEST STAR SHIMMERS IN THE BLACK SKY. NO ONE CAN SEE IT, BUT IT'S THERE.

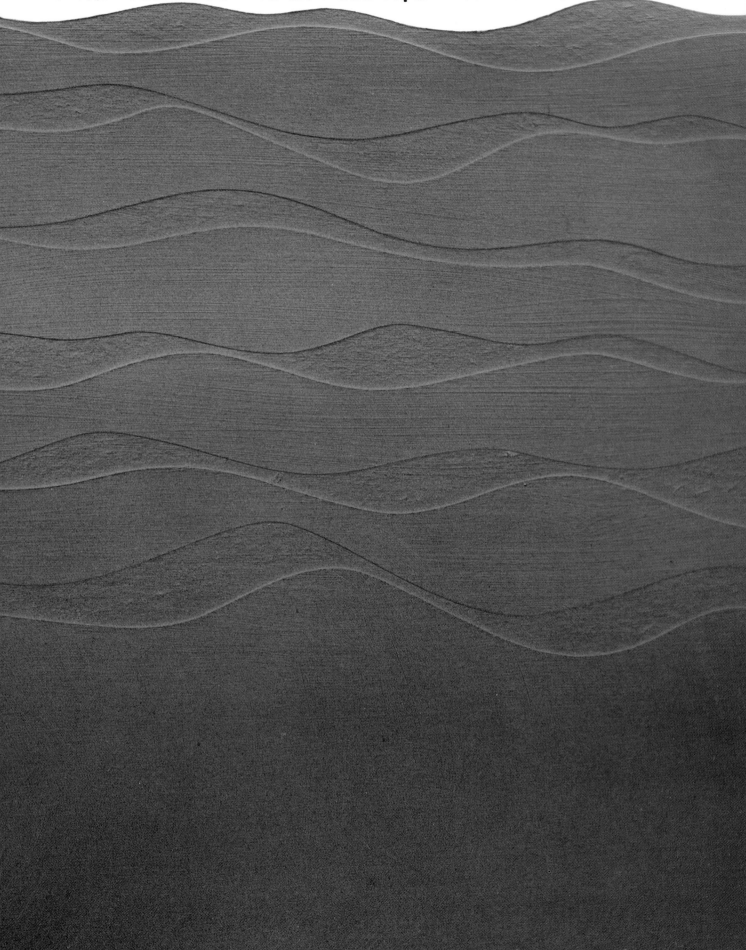

AND SNUG AS A SECRET, IN THE WARMTH OF YOUR MOTHER'S WOMB, YOU WERE THERE.
A PROTECTIVE SAC, FILLED WITH WATER, FORMED AROUND YOU. INSIDE YOUR SAC YOU WERE SO TINY, SO STILL, NO ONE KNEW ABOUT YOU.

EXCEPT GOD.

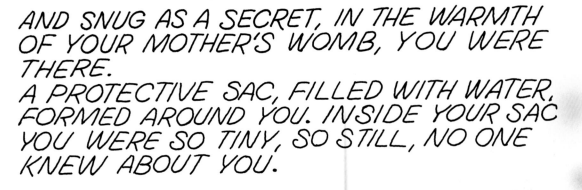

AT THE MOMENT YOUR LIFE BEGAN,
EVERYTHING WAS THERE THAT WOULD
MAKE YOU THE SPECIAL PERSON YOU ARE.
ALREADY GOD   KNEW WHETHER YOU
WOULD BE A   BOY OR A GIRL, WHAT
COLOR HAIR AND EYES YOU WOULD HAVE,
AND HOW TALL YOU WOULD BECOME.
AND AT THE CENTER OF THIS LIFE WAS
YOUR SOUL, WHICH WAS CREATED WITH ALL
THE JOY AND GLORY OF GOD'S LOVE,
BECAUSE HE WANTED YOU.

YOUR BODY WAS SEPARATE FROM YOUR MOTHER'S BODY, BUT YOU NEEDED HER TO HELP YOU GROW. SO A CORD FORMED FROM YOUR BODY TO HERS, AND THROUGH THAT CORD CAME THE NOURISHMENT FROM HER BODY TO YOURS.

IN FOUR WEEKS YOU GREW TO BE ONE-FOURTH INCH LONG, AS CURLED AS THE SWIRL IN A GLEAMING TURBAN SHELL. YOU HAD A ROUND HEAD, AS BIG AS HALF YOUR BODY, AND A HEART THAT BEAT WITH NO MORE SOUND THAN A WHISPER. YOUR ARMS AND LEGS WERE BEGINNING TO FORM, AND YOU HAD A MOUTH.

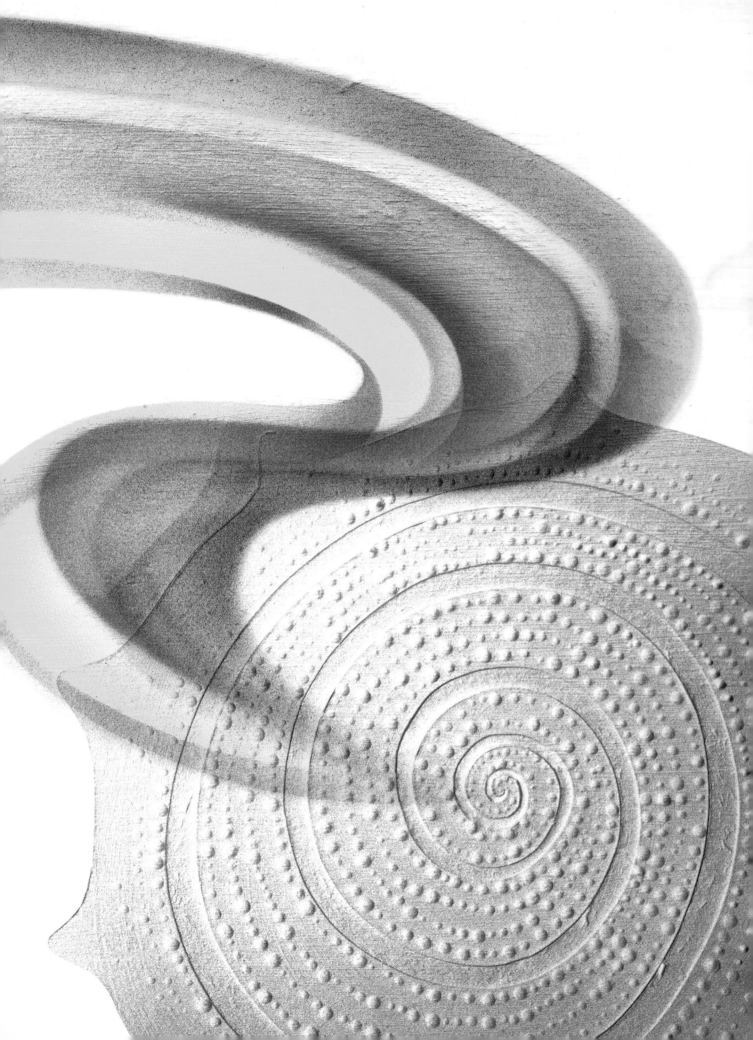

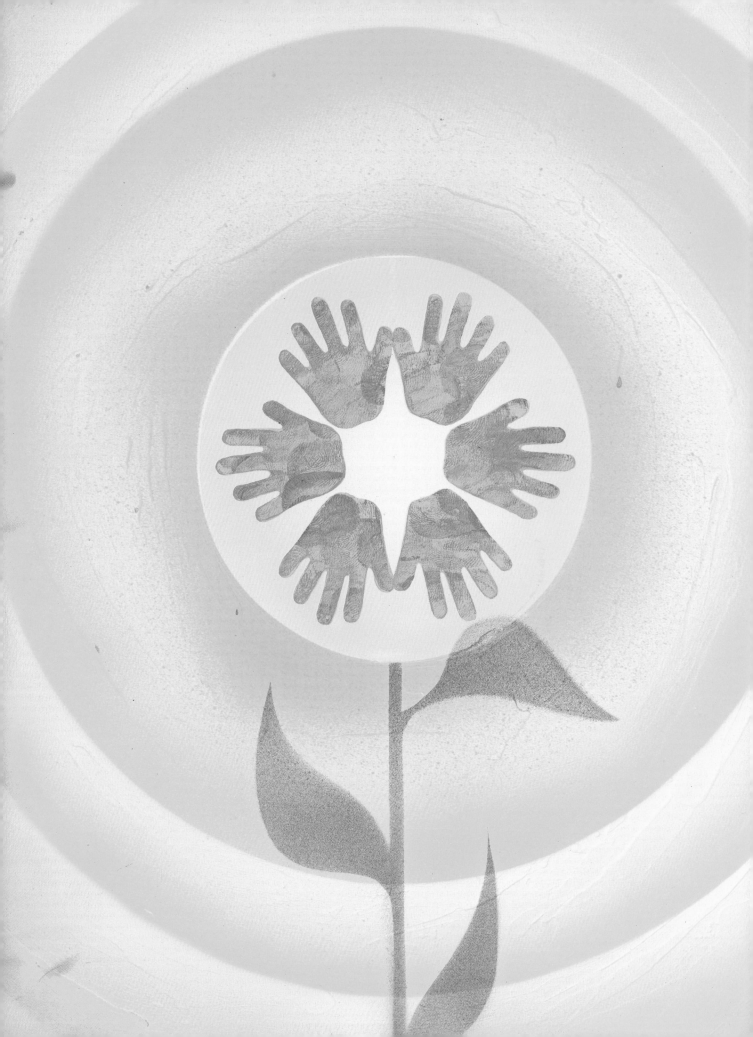

BY THE END OF YOUR SIXTH WEEK OF LIFE YOUR BRAIN HAD DEVELOPED ENOUGH TO SEND OUT BRAIN WAVES THAT SHOWED IT WAS LIVING AND ACTIVE. AND SOMETIMES, IN THE SOFT, WARM CUSHION WHERE YOU LIVED, YOU MOVED--LITTLE, QUIET MOVEMENTS, NOT STRONG ENOUGH YET FOR YOUR MOTHER TO FEEL.

YOUR BODY WAS NOURISHED BY YOUR MOTHER'S BODY, AND YOU GREW. WHEN YOU WERE TWO MONTHS OLD YOU WERE NOT MUCH MORE THAN ONE INCH LONG; BUT YOU HAD A FACE, WITH EYES, EARS, AND A NOSE. YOU HAD HANDS AND FEET; AND THE FINGERS WHICH WERE FORMING ALREADY HAD THE FINGERPRINTS THAT WOULD BE YOURS, AND ONLY YOURS, FOR THE REST OF YOUR LIFE.

BY NOW YOUR PARENTS KNEW ABOUT YOU AND SHARED THIS GLADNESS.

ALL YOUR ENERGIES WENT INTO THE JOB OF GROWING, AND AT YOUR THIRD MONTH OF LIFE INSIDE THE WOMB YOU WERE THREE INCHES LONG. YOU HAD EYELIDS, THINNER THAN BUTTERFLY WINGS, THAT STAYED SOFTLY CLOSED OVER YOUR EYES. AND YOU HAD TINY FINGERNAILS AND TOENAILS. YOU COULD SWALLOW, AND YOU MOVED MORE EASILY IN YOUR WATER-FILLED SAC THAT GREW LARGER AS YOU GREW LARGER.

IN ANOTHER FOUR WEEKS YOU HAD
DOUBLED YOUR SIZE.

AT FOUR MONTHS   OF LIFE YOUR
BONES WERE STRONGER, AND NOW--
FOR THE FIRST TIME--YOUR MOTHER
MIGHT HAVE FELT YOU STRETCH OUT
AN ARM AND PULL IT BACK.
YOU COULD KICK YOUR LEGS AND TURN
YOUR HEAD.

BUT WHEN YOU
RESTED YOU CURLED
COMFORTABLY INTO
THE DARK WARMTH,
WITH YOUR KNEES PULLED
UP AND YOUR ANKLES
CROSSED, AND YOUR ARMS
FOLDED IN FRONT OF YOUR FACE.

YOUR HEART WAS STRONG ENOUGH FOR THE
DOCTOR TO HEAR IT THROUGH HIS STETHOSCOPE
WHEN YOU WERE FIVE MONTHS OLD. MAYBE HE
ASKED YOUR MOTHER IF SHE, TOO, WOULD LIKE TO
LISTEN THROUGH THE STETHOSCOPE TO THIS TINY
PERSON GROWING INSIDE HER BODY.
YOU WERE NOW ABOUT NINE INCHES LONG AND
WEIGHED ALMOST ELEVEN OUNCES. LONG AGO
YOUR BABY TEETH HAD FORMED UNDER YOUR
GUMS, AND NOW YOUR PERMANENT TEETH
WERE FORMING. SOFT HAIR WAS GROWING ON
YOUR HEAD.

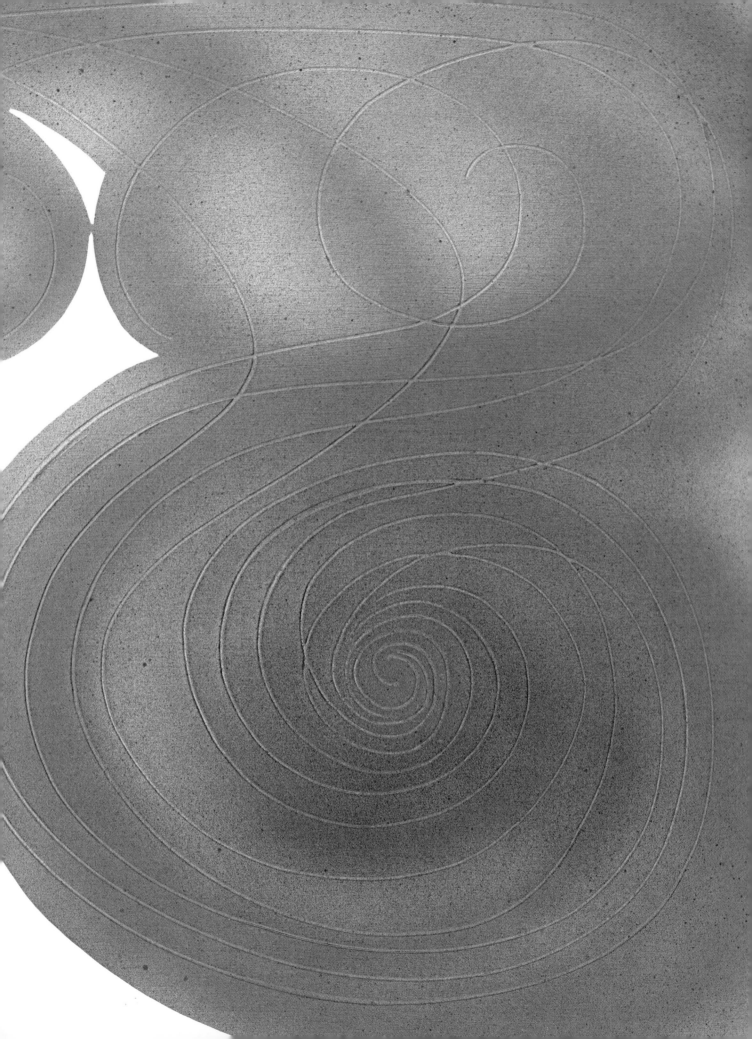

STILL YOU GREW, AND YOUR WATER SAC AND THE
WOMB STRETCHED AND GREW LARGER, TOO.
SOMETIMES YOUR MOTHER COULD FEEL YOU
MOVING AND PUSHING AGAINST THE
WALLS AROUND YOU. AND MAYBE
YOU COULD SENSE HER
HAPPINESS AS SHE
KNEW YOU WERE THERE
AND LOVED YOU.

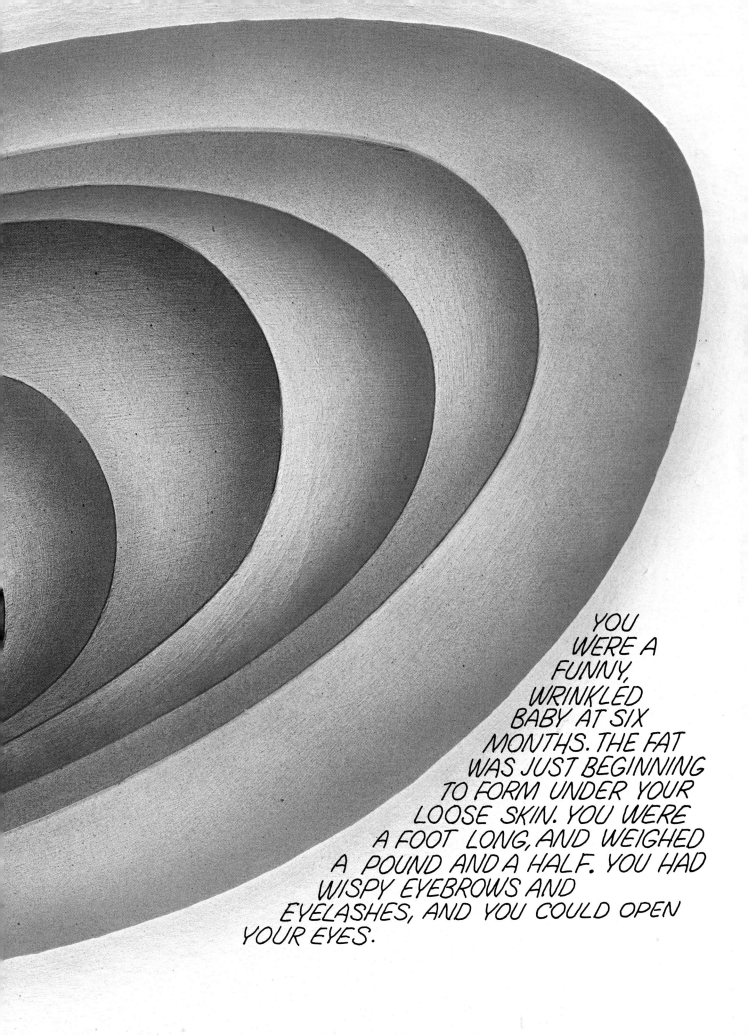

YOU WERE A FUNNY, WRINKLED BABY AT SIX MONTHS. THE FAT WAS JUST BEGINNING TO FORM UNDER YOUR LOOSE SKIN. YOU WERE A FOOT LONG, AND WEIGHED A POUND AND A HALF. YOU HAD WISPY EYEBROWS AND EYELASHES, AND YOU COULD OPEN YOUR EYES.

IN THE SOOTHING COMFORT OF YOUR OWN QUIET WORLD YOU SUCKED YOUR THUMB. BUT WHEN YOU HICCUPPED YOU WEREN'T QUIET AT ALL, AND YOUR MOTHER COULD FEEL YOU **JUMPING** AND **BUMPING** INSIDE HER.

SHE COULD FEEL YOU ROLL AND TURN
EVEN MORE STRONGLY WHEN YOU HAD
LIVED FOR SEVEN MONTHS, BECAUSE YOU
WERE NOW FOURTEEN INCHES LONG, AND
YOUR WEIGHT WAS TWO-AND-A-HALF
POUNDS. ALL THE ORGANS OF
YOUR BODY HAD DEVELOPED INTO
WHAT THEY SHOULD BE. BUT IN THE
WARMTH OF YOUR PROTECTED GROWING
PLACE YOU WERE STILL NOT QUITE
STRONG ENOUGH, NOT QUITE READY
TO BE BORN.

YOU EXERCISED IN THE WOMB, A BUSY
ACTIVE BABY. YOU WERE NOURISHED
AND YOU GREW PLUMPER. YOU WERE
HELPING IN EVERY WAY YOU
COULD TO BE READY FOR YOUR
LIFE AFTER BIRTH. YOU WERE
EIGHT MONTHS OLD NOW,
LONGER AND **HEAVIER**
AND **STRONGER**.

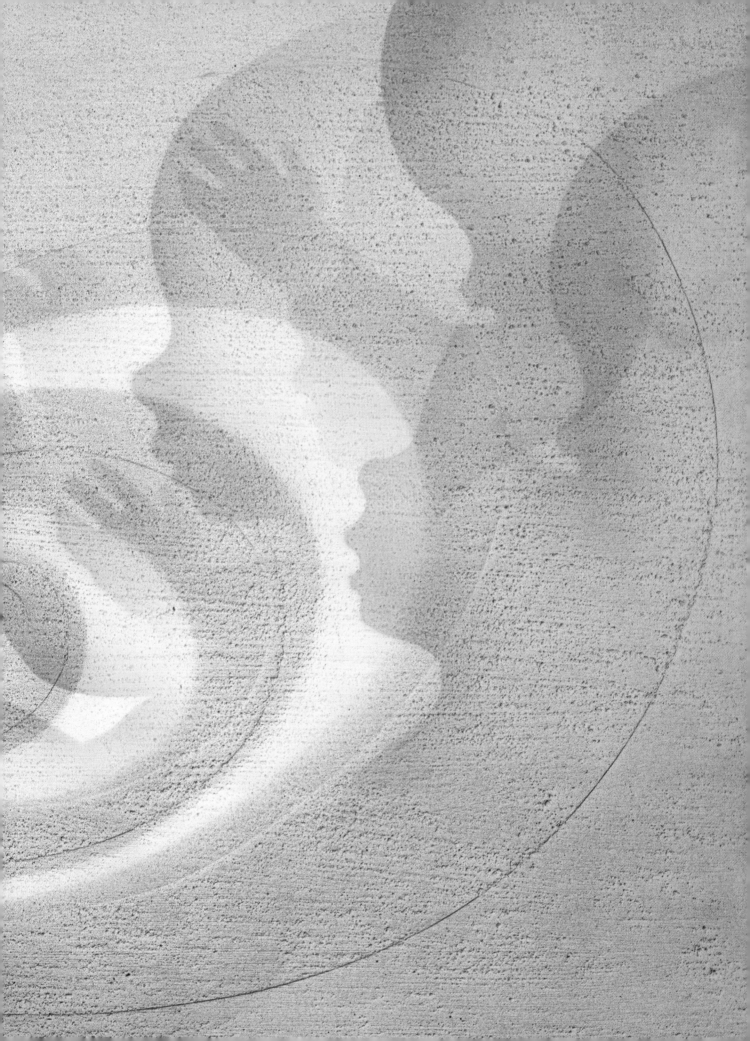

DURING THE NINTH MONTH OF YOUR LIFE BEFORE YOU WERE BORN, YOU GREW TO THE LENGTH AND WEIGHT YOU WOULD HAVE AT BIRTH. MAYBE YOU WERE NINETEEN INCHES LONG, MAYBE TWENTY-TWO. YOU MIGHT HAVE WEIGHED SIX POUNDS, MAYBE NINE, MAYBE SOMEWHERE IN THE MIDDLE. YOU WERE PLUMP, AND YOUR SKIN WASN'T AS WRINKLED OR RED. THE HAIR ON YOUR HEAD WAS THICKER, AND YOUR EYELASHES CURLED AGAINST YOUR ROUND CHEEKS.

NOW YOU
WERE CROWDED
IN YOUR WATER SAC,
WITH YOUR KNEES PULLED UP
AGAINST YOUR CHEST AND
YOUR HEAD BENT DOWN.
IT WAS HARD FOR
YOU TO MOVE AS
MUCH AS YOU
HAD BEFORE.

AT SOME MOMENT YOUR BODY AND YOUR MOTHER'S BODY KNEW IT WAS TIME FOR YOU TO BE BORN, AND THE WALLS OF THE WOMB SQUEEZED AGAINST YOU. THEY PUSHED YOU HEADFIRST THROUGH THE PASSAGEWAY IN YOUR MOTHER'S BODY, OUT OF YOUR WARM, WET, COMFORTABLE GROWING PLACE.

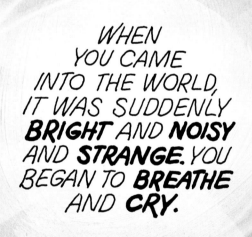

WHEN YOU CAME INTO THE WORLD, IT WAS SUDDENLY **BRIGHT** AND **NOISY** AND **STRANGE.** YOU BEGAN TO **BREATHE** AND **CRY.**

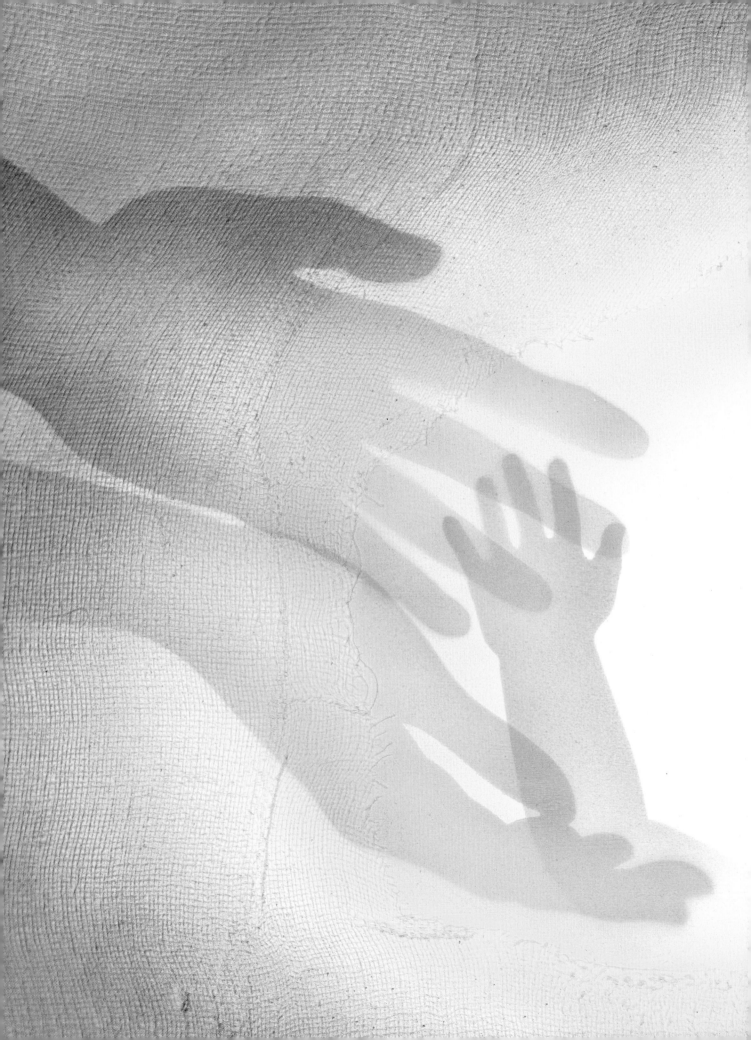

YOUR MOTHER EAGERLY REACHED OUT HER ARMS TO HOLD YOU. ALTHOUGH THIS WORLD WAS NEW TO YOU, YOUR MOTHER'S LOVE AND STEADILY BEATING HEART WERE FAMILIAR AND COMFORTING. YOU COULD NOT TAKE CARE OF YOURSELF NOW ANY MORE THAN YOU COULD BEFORE YOU WERE BORN, BUT THIS DID NOT WORRY YOU, BECAUSE YOUR MOTHER WAS THERE.

AND YOUR WORLD OF LOVE WAS LARGER. YOU FELT THE STRONG ARMS OF YOUR FATHER AND, WITH YOUR FUZZY NEW EYESIGHT, SAW THE SMILES OF OTHERS WHO LOVED YOU AND WOULD HELP TO CARE FOR YOU.

BUT NOW THAT YOU HAD COME INTO THIS NEW WORLD, YOU WERE TIRED, AND YOU SLEPT. MAYBE YOU DREAMED ABOUT THE SNUG, QUIET PLACE WHERE YOUR LIFE BEGAN. MAYBE YOU DREAMED OF THE GENTLE ROCKING OF THAT WATERY SAC AND THE STEADY BEAT OF YOUR MOTHER'S HEART.

AND MAYBE YOU DREAMED OF GOD,
WHO SO VERY LONG AGO HAD
DREAMED OF YOU.